3

STRATEGIES

OF

MANAGING STRESS

Dr. PASINDU ABEYSUNDARA

(MBBS-SRI LANKA)

The information provided in this book is designed to complement but not replace, the relationship between a patient and his/her physician. Any person above age 18 can use this information unless it has a very serious health concern.

Moreover, the information provided here should not be used over the professional opinion of the own physician of a patient with a particular illness that needs a continual and follow-up treatment for that illness although the information provided here may aid in the management of that illness directly or indirectly.

Table of Contents

Introduction

In this modern world, as a person, or as a society, people are running after their goals and their dreams. They tend to chase after those dreams, forgetting themselves and their loved ones. Some people chase after money while others run for fame, power, and so on. But no one seems to be running after the happiness, love, forgiveness….

What could these lives bring to them? Are they achieving what they want? Maybe not. When we look at the lives of these busy people, what we see is desperation, unhappiness, greediness. Are they happy? Certainly not. What they surely have are depression, anxiety, mental stress, anger, and so on.

As a result of these busy lifestyles, piled up unresolved business at the workplace, children, exam stress, etc. and so many other physical, mental and other social stresses surround each one of us.

We can take one person as an example. It's you. Are you overwhelmed? Do the things are not happening in your favor at the moment? Are you feeling angry about something? Are you feeling stressed and feel like "I need a break"? Then this is for you!

What is stress?

Stress is a physiological response that elicits from our body when we face a difficult situation. In the normal evolutionary process, the man had to fight with animals to stay strong and survive. Hence, there are a few stress hormones evolved to cope up with this stressful environment that would let us handle the situation.

For instance, imagine a fierce animal is following you! The first thing you feel would be to run for your life. Some hormones like cortisol, adrenaline act on our systems of the body to elicit this response.

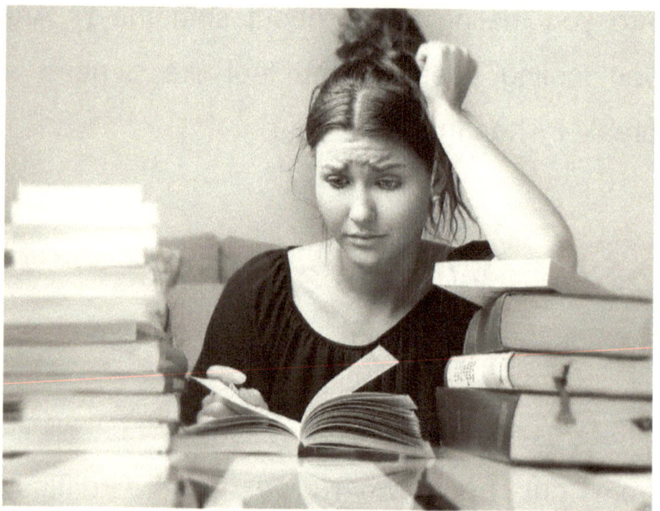

Studying for exams can cause mental stress

What are the Effects of Longtime exposure to Stress?

However, like a normal person, we may need this stress response to do our day to day work properly. It may give us the driving force to achieve certain goals in our life.

For instance, if you are studying for an exam, the stress of knowing the exam is on the scheduled day will drive you to make a plan and study properly to pass the exam. Hence, having a little bit of stress is acceptable to run our normal day to day lives.

On the other hand, what will happen if we face stressful situations for a long time? That's when your body adapts to that stress in an unwanted fashion leading to major health hazards.

Certainly, as you expose to long term stress, scientists found that there are numerous changes occur within our body. Your white blood cell production reduces. This, in turn, inhibits the inflammatory response against bacteria and viruses leading your immune system to shut down. Therefore, you are susceptible to other disease conditions as well.

Other than that, it accelerates the clogging of your blood vessels leading you to have heart attacks and strokes. And your brain cells get smaller and they lose intercellular connections so your mental functions especially learning and memorizing skills will deteriorate with time.

Another one important effect of long-term stress is that it can cause gastrointestinal problems like losing the appetite, stomach ulcers, and poor absorption of nutrients from the gut wall, etc.

Similarly, long-term stress can affect your endocrine system. For instance, if a lady is facing a stressful situation, she may not experience her normal regular menstrual cycles thus she may not be able to get pregnant timely. Not only these effects but also researchers found that long term stress might induce cancers as well.

Strategy No.1
Understanding the Cause and Effect

This strategy is based on understanding the cause of your stress and then eliminating the cause. Therefore, you will ultimately eliminate the bad effects of stress.

For this to happen, you should have a calm and quiet mind, and preferably a calm environment too. You can follow these steps when you are stressed.

Understand what is the Root Cause of the Stress

When you are under stress, the first thing you have to do is to take a deep breath and sit in someplace comfortably and think what is the root cause that makes you stress out.

It could be a financial problem, it could be piled up unresolved business work, it could be an exam, it could be another function that you have to attend which you don't have time available to attend to.

But, whatever the problem, if you **identify the root cause** then there will be a solution.

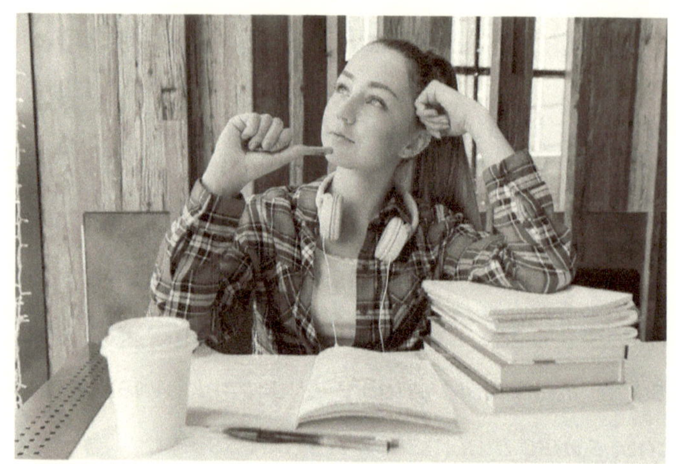

Sit in a calm and quiet place and think of the
root cause for the problem

Work out the Solution to your Problem

Once you identify your problem or problems,
you have to think of logical ways of eliminating
that problem.

For example, if you are having lots of
unresolved business work at your workplace,

you should think of logical ways how to finish off those work.

First, **list down all the work you have to do**. Then in front of each task, write down when is the deadline that you should finish that task. After that write how many days or how many hours left for you to finish that task in front.

By doing this, automatically you will get a task sheet telling you which work is to be done first and which should be done next. Most importantly, this will give you an idea of **prioritizing your work**.

Once you finish each work, tick off or cut it off. When you finish one or two tasks, you will feel the thrill, and you will feel the rush. And your brain will tell you, "let's do this", and "let's do that", and you will get the driving force and motivation.

When you come across an easy task and a difficult task, first finish the easy task quickly and then concentrate on the difficult one. In this way, several small tasks will be all done, and you will be left with a few bigger tasks only.

Besides, while you are doing an important task, someone might need you to divert your effort to another less important task. **Learn to say NO** to them. If you don't put your effort to finish important tasks timely manner, you will likely have mental stress again.

Use other Supportive ways of Relieving Stress

While you are engaging in your work, there are other supportive ways of relieving stress.

Some people find it **listening to their favorite singer,** or **listening to classical music** would relieve the stress.

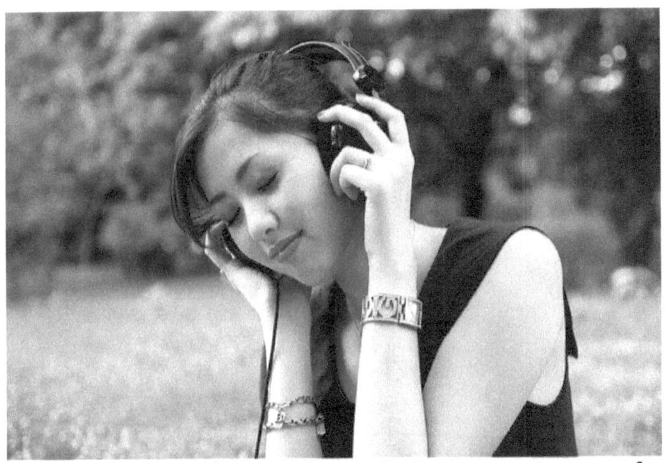

Listening to classical music is a great way of relieving stress

Similarly, some find it in some rituals, like eating their favorite food, **drinking a hot tea/coffee,** or **smelling their favorite scent,** etc.

However, there is a science behind this as well. Sensory nerve endings responsible for sensing smell are connected to the brain in humans where the brain regulates our cortisol level. So, scientists think that this can have an association to reduce stress with these senses.

Another important point to emphasize is that **spending time in nature** is a great way of relieving stress too. Going out to a park, or keeping fresh flowers in your room will help you a lot in relieving stress.

Change your Lifestyle Patterns

If you are staying in the office for all 24 hours without going out with friends, or family, you are more likely to have long term stress.

When we **make out with our loved ones,** we feel attached, bonded, secured feelings that in turn would raise a hormone called "oxytocin" in the body. This hormone is responsible to relieve stress.

So, throw out a party once in a while. Laugh a little bit. Go to a family dinner. Play with your children, or play out with your puppy, or dog. These simple things will relieve your stress a great deal.

Moreover, try to **cut down alcohol, and stop smoking.** These are also positive lifestyle changes that can alleviate stress. For instance, if you are studying for an exam usage of alcohol might reduce your concentrating ability leading you to stress out.

Do some **regular exercises** like cycling, swimming, jogging, etc. If you are physically fit, all your systems of the body are healthy so you are less likely to get mental stress as well.

In conclusion,

To sum up, strategy number 1 of managing mental stress is not that difficult to implement. All you need to do is to identify the root cause of your problems and start finding solutions.

Strategy No.2 Practicing Mindfulness

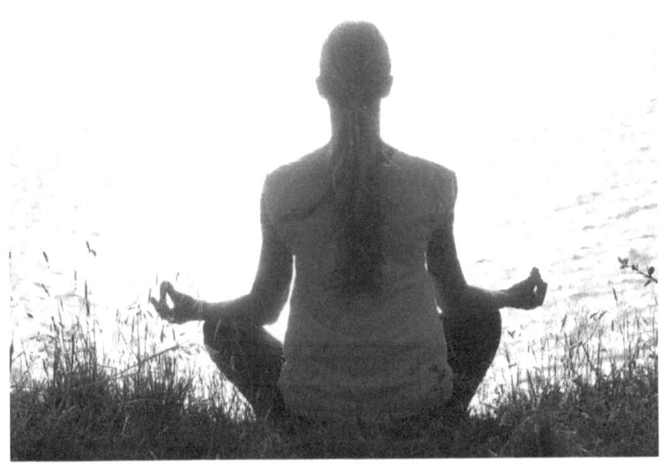

Practicing mindfulness is one of the widely researched subjects in the western world for the last few decades. Whereas, the roots of this subject are well-known core teachings in Buddhism in the eastern world.

However, the overall message to the world is very fruitful in many ways. Not only it helps an individual with its physical and mental health benefits, but also it benefits interpersonal relationships as well.

What is Mindfulness?

According to the researchers, mindfulness is a psychological state of awareness and a mode of processing information with certain practices that promote the aforementioned awareness.

In other words, they define mindfulness as a state of psychological freedom that occurs when attention remains quiet and limber without attachment to any particular point of view.

Simply, we can extract this and say mindfulness is having a *moment by moment awareness of one's experience without judgment*. In Buddhism, the Pali word "sati" refers to a similar state like mindfulness. Broadly, it refers to awareness, attention, and remembering.

Importance of Mindfulness

Nowadays, everybody is overwhelmed, feels out of control and they say that they are depressed, or anxious. People worry about the incidents that happened in the past or they worry thinking about the incidents that may take place in the future.

Most of them are driven by their emotions, and a lot of them are suffering from mental illnesses like depression, anxiety, etc.

For example, how many of us have sat in front of the television and watched it while taking our meals not knowing what we have eaten, or not enjoying the taste of that meal, or the refreshing smell of that meal?

How many of us have used social media on our mobile phones without knowing what happens in the surroundings?

The ultimate result is that we don't satisfy ourselves, and run behind the stressors of life making our lives more vulnerable.

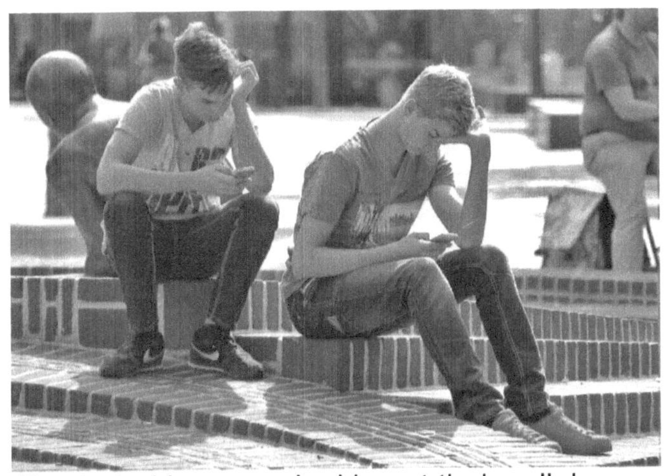

Frustrated boys are looking at their cellphones not knowing anything about their surroundings

Mindfulness is a way of learning how to accept and work with your mind, yourself, and others.

Further, it is about accepting your life circumstances discovering the joy in everyday moments.

Cultivating Mindfulness

There are many ways to cultivate mindfulness.

In ancient India, a character named *"Patanjali"* had founded Yoga. Practicing Yoga is a great way of practicing mindfulness as altogether it covers the body, spirit, and the intellect of an individual. He named these as "Yoga Sutras".

Similarly, *"Tai Chi"* which was originated in China is also a great way of practicing mindfulness.

However, in this second strategy of managing stress, we will discuss practicing mindfulness meditation as a way of cultivating mindfulness.

To easily understand the concepts of mindfulness, firstly we can take a look at Buddhist teachings on mindfulness.

Disclaimer

It is very important to emphasize that although people worship it as a religion, Buddhism is not a religion. It is more of a philosophy. If you are a Christian, or a Muslim, or worshipping any other respectful religion, you should not need to become a Buddhist to take and understand some of the governing principles of Buddhism.

The purpose of the following section of this book is to give you a good understanding of how mindfulness and mindfulness meditation can be practiced by a person to manage stress and to get away from other feelings of negative thoughts, anger, depression, and so on.

Buddhist Teachings on Practicing Mindfulness Meditation

Mindfulness meditation is synonymous to the "*Vipassana*" meditation taught in the Theravada Buddhism. "*Vipassana*" in Pali means "Insight" or having a clear awareness. It is a form of meditation that is designed to gradually develop the mindfulness.

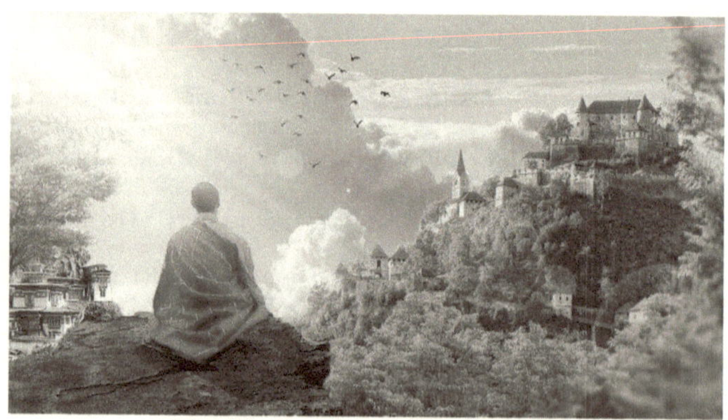
Meditating Buddhist monk

"*Ti-lakkhana*" – the Three Characteristics of Existence

Among the Lord Buddha's teachings, there is a concept called "*ti-lakkhana*" with three important doctrines "*Anicca*", "*Dukkha*", and "*Anatta*" which are the three "marks" or basic characteristics of all phenomenal existence.

First, "*Anicca*" explains that all the beings and non-beings in the world are impermanent. They will arise and pass out but nothing will last forever.

Secondly, "*Dukkha*" explains that dissatisfaction, disease, stress, and/or suffering. Nothing in the physical world can bring permanent satisfaction to anyone.

Lastly, "*Anatta*" explains that there is in humans no permanent, underlying substance that can be called the soul. Every pleasant or unpleasant experience you face happens independently from you whether you like it or not.

For example,

Everybody has hair on their heads. It does not last forever. Your hair may be beautiful at present but it changes its color when you grow old. It may fall off. No matter how hard you try to keep it in the shape, it changes. That is the "*anicca*" quality of hair.

Similarly, the person who bears the hair has to cut it when it grows. He has to treat diseases like dandruff, headlice, etc. You have to comb it every morning to keep its shape. And all these things make the owner suffer because of the hair. That is the "*dukkha*" quality of hair.

Further, though you try everything to keep it black, it becomes white when you get older. Although you try different methods, it may fall off from the head with time. These things happen whether you like it or not. That is the *"anatta"* quality of hair.

Likewise, Buddhism explains that these three marks are universal to anyone or anything.

In *"Vipassana"* meditation, the person systemically cultivates mindfulness by applying these three principles to the four main foundations; his bodily sensations, emotions, thoughts or the consciousness, and *"Dharma"*, which is the law of nature or the surrounding environment.

The "*Satipatthana Sutta*"

This is the text that contains the Lord Buddha's teachings on practicing mindfulness meditation. It is thought to be the foundation for the modern concepts of mindfulness meditation.

A biologist Professor Jon Kabat Zinn was heavily influenced by these teachings as a student. And later he pioneered a new approach to treat people living with chronic illnesses with a stress reduction program based on mindfulness.

This approach is now practiced all over the world as Mindfulness-Based Stress Reduction (MBSR). A lot of researchers found that MBSR is very effective in treating people with stress, depression, anxiety, and even high blood pressure.

In the *"Satipatthana Sutta"*, Lord Buddha explains four main foundations of practicing mindfulness meditation. They are bodily sensations, Feelings, Thoughts, or Consciousness, and *"Dharma"*.

1. Bodily Sensations.

Mindful people develop an awareness of their posture and the bodily movements and sensations as well as their breathing patterns.

They recognize the *"anicca"* quality of the body and consider the body is not a permanent thing, and it is merely a vehicle that they happen to be inhabiting. Further, they do not attach to these bodily sensations as they recognize these are due to the *"Anatta"* quality of the body.

2. Feelings

Mindful people develop an awareness of their feelings. They recognize that there are happy feelings, and there are sad feelings. They don't attach to those feelings as they keep watching them come and go.

Moreover, they develop the understanding that all emotions are transient, and they also have the aforementioned qualities of *"ti-lakkhana"*.

3. Thoughts, or Consciousness

Mindful people develop an awareness of their thoughts. When they get thoughts like greediness, desire, hate, ignorance, etc. they quickly recognize the qualities of *"ti-lakkhana"* of their thoughts, and they understand them as mere thoughts. They don't attach to those thoughts or consciousness.

4. *"Dharma"*

Mindful people develop the awareness about the law of nature or the surrounding environment as described from Sanskrit word "Dharma". This is a complex concept in Buddhism which needs care, and well-committed training to fully understand. However, understanding this would lead to an understanding of the four noble truths in Buddhism.

As we discussed in the above context, by practicing mindfulness meditation, or the *"Vipassana"* meditation, a person can systemically cultivate mindfulness by applying these principles of *"Ti-lakkhana"*, to the aforementioned four main foundations.

By practicing mindfulness meditation, a person can not only achieve physical fitness but also mental health benefits like interpersonal, intrapersonal, and emotional benefits. We will discuss these benefits in the following section.

Emotional Benefits of Practicing Mindfulness Meditation

It Helps to Regulate your Emotions Effectively

The research found out that people who undergo mindfulness meditation **enhances their attention and concentration.** Similarly, it **enhances their working memory capacity** as well. This would lead them to find effective emotions regulating strategies like handling mental stress.

According to a study, they showed sad movies to a group of people who practiced MBSR for 8 weeks and to another control group. The result was that the anxiety, depression and somatic distress was less in the group of people who practiced MBSR compared to the other group.

This shows that practicing mindfulness meditation shifts a person's ability to employ emotions differently, and the emotions they experience may be processed by their brains differently.

Likewise, several other studies found that people who are practicing mindfulness meditation elicit positive emotions, minimize negative emotions, & rumination too.

It Helps to Focus the Attention and Suppress Distressing Information

Researchers found that people who are practicing mindfulness meditation can focus their attention on the cognitive task at hand effectively. Cognitive tasks refer to the day to day mental tasks we will have to do.

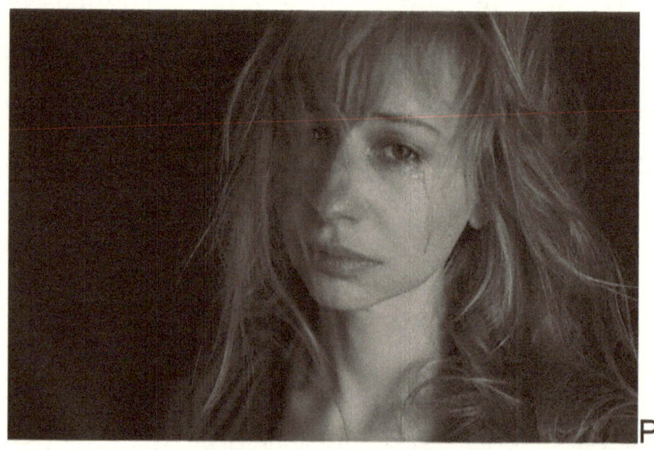

Practicing mindfulness meditation help people to disengage from emotionally unpleasant or upsetting stimuli

Furthermore, it can help people to disengage from emotionally unpleasant, or upsetting stimuli. Thus, for a mindful person, the death of a loved one may not cause much distress as it would do to a normal person!

Intrapersonal Benefits of Practicing Mindfulness Meditation

It Promotes Self-insight, Morality, and Intuition

By practicing mindfulness meditation, one develops the awareness of all the feelings and thoughts in day to day activities, etc. Thus, they will enhance their ability to understand what is right, and what is wrong. This makes a better person who doesn't attach to the everyday stressors of life.

It Promotes Increased Information Processing Speed

As the mindful person enhances his attention, and memory capacity, they can process more information at a given time. Needless to say, this is very important to students as they need to retain information, and to learn something quickly. Moreover, they are likely to perform well in the classroom when compared to normal students.

It Improves one's Empathy, Compassion, and Certain other Skills

By practicing mindfulness meditation, people tend to look more constructively upon the problems they face. This makes them compare that the other person is also another human being who has struggles in their lives like them. This non-judging behavior improves their compassion and empathy towards other people.

Research says that healthcare workers who undergo MBSR elicited more compassion and empathy towards their clients. Further, they reported that they feel more connected to their clients, and feel their sufferings when treating their clients.

Certainly, this is a piece of great news for the psychotherapists, doctors, nurses, etc. as this can improve the connection between them and their clients. On the other hand, mental health counselors can improve their skills of connecting with their patients by practicing mindfulness meditation too.

Decreases Stress, Anxiety and Rumination

Studies showed that the medical students and nursing students who undergo MBSR, experience less stress, & anxiety, less fatigue & rumination when compared to normal people. Similarly, they showed more positive thoughts, and less negative mood too when compared to normal people.

That is why they use MBSR techniques in almost everywhere in the world as a method of relieving stress.

Practicing Mindfulness Meditation Increases your Physical Health and Wellness

Research says that MBSR can reduce your risk from getting cardiovascular disease, reduce high blood pressure, reduce chronic pain, and improve sleep.

Likewise, it can improve your immune function so you will be healthy from a lot of ailments too.

Interpersonal Benefits of Practicing Mindfulness Meditation

Not only it helps a person to enhance their inner powers but also it helps a person to improve his relationships as well.

By practicing mindfulness meditation, a person trains himself to respond to a situation in a non-attached, and non-judgmental way. Therefore, when he faces a problem in his relationship, he responds constructively respecting others' emotions too.

Certainly, this is a very important thing to continue a healthy relationship. Furthermore, this leads to increased relationship satisfaction so the married couples are more likely to stay together in their lifetime.

Above all, a mindful person is more likely to act in social situations with responsibility, and with clarity of mind. This may lead them to become team leaders in peer groups as well.

A simple way to Start.....

At first, practicing mindfulness meditation may look difficult. It certainly is. According to Buddhism, a person must start meditation minute by minute daily, and increase the time day by day. It needs your commitment, to achieve the above benefits we discussed above.

However, you can start to be mindful when you are doing small day to day chores. Think that I'm doing this thing now. And keep your mind on the work you are doing at the moment. If you happen to be thinking about another thing, refocus your mind on the task at hand.

You can start this soon after you get up from your night's sleep. Mindfully do all the work. Simply think, I'm brushing my teeth now. I'm eating breakfast now. What I'm eating for breakfast? Likewise.

Believe me! If you do all your chores with mindfulness, in the afternoon, or night, you will be able to **_recall all the actions_** you did from the morning to the time you are recalling, one by one!

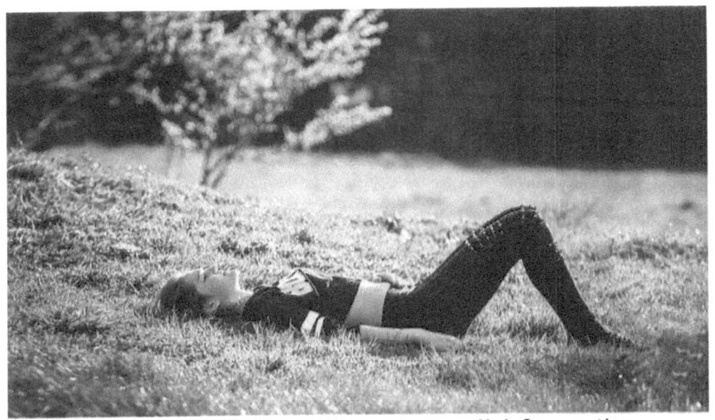

Think about the things you did from the morning to the evening. If you did all the tasks mindfully, you will be able to recall the things you did.

What to do Next?

Starting Mindfulness Meditation – The Early Stages

Before starting mindfulness meditation, it is advisable to practice mindfulness in your day to day work at least, and then develop some ability to concentrate your thoughts in one place.

In Buddhism, Lord Buddha had instructed his disciples to do *"Samatha"* meditation, for example, loving-kindness meditation, before starting *"Vipassana"* meditation so they can achieve calmness of mind beforehand.

However, when you achieve some sort of mindfulness, you can practice mindfulness meditation. Here, the starting point is to concentrate on your breathing patterns and develop awareness.

Breathing Exercise...

Firstly, go to a calm, and quiet place. This could be a separate area in your garden or a separate room in your house. The idea is to stay away from distractions and maintain silence while you are meditating.

As a beginner, some people find it easy to develop mental concentration when there is absolute silence. Conversely, if you can't find a place with complete silence, you can enjoy a calm, and quiet place with some privacy. That would do.

Then, sit in a way crossing your legs tucked in, holding your back erect though not strained, or rigid. One has to maintain a proper posture to practice this meditation as all the bones of the spine are linked together in an erect position.

The hands should be placed gently on the lap both palms facing upwards, the back of the right hand over the palm of the left hand. The head should be held straight, tilted a slight angle downwards, the nose perpendicular to the novel. The eyes can be closed softly, or even half-closed depending on the way which is more comfortable for you.

Now, you have to keep your concentration on the tip of your nose. This will be the main focus of your attention in this meditation. You should be mindful of the place where the incoming breath and outgoing breath passes through this area like a gatekeeper watching over a gate observing who is getting in, and who is getting out.

Now, you should be mindful when you are breathing in, and out. If you happen to breathe in a long breath, you have to comprehend this with full awareness. Similarly, if you breathe out a long breath, you have to comprehend this with full awareness. On the other hand, if you breathe in a short breath, you have to comprehend this with full awareness, and if you breathe out a short breath, you have to comprehend this with full awareness.

Another important point to emphasize is that you should never try to control the breathing pattern, or hold back your breath with conscious effort as this can make you fatigued, and break your mental concentration, and awareness.

Just maintain the mindfulness naturally at the tip of your nose where the in-breaths, out-breaths are felt entering and leaving the nostrils.

What if you are distracted?

This is when counting comes into the act. When you fix your attention at the tip of the nose when the breath-in enters, and then the breath-out leaves the tip of the nose, this is considered a one. There are a few methods of counting. The easiest is as follows;

The first breath felt is counted as "one, one"; the second as "two, two"; the third as "three, three"; and so on. Likewise, you should count up to the tenth breath which is counted as "ten, ten." Then you should return to "one, one" and continue again up to "ten, ten." This is repeated over and over from one to ten.

Most importantly, you should understand that mere counting is not useful. You should always keep you focus on your breath as a gatekeeper watches over the people coming in, and out passing the gate. Counting is an easy method to control the wandering mind. If by chance, you happen to miss the count, this means that your mind has lost its focus. Start counting from one again, and continue. In the beginning, you may lose the count thousands of times, but with time, and with practice, you will improve.

As the practice develops, there may come a time when the in-breathing and out-breathing take a shorter course, and it is not possible to count the same number many times. If this occurs, then you have to count quickly "one," "two," "three," etc. When you count in this manner, you can comprehend the difference between a long in-breath, and out-breath, and a short in-breath and out-breath with awareness.

These are the early stages of mindfulness meditation. You can follow these steps easily in the home environment too. But keep in mind that it is not that easy to implement these practices if you don't devote yourself to them. However, with commitment, if you practice this, the outcome will be fruitful.

NOTE - The above meditation exercise is based on the early stages of the "*Ana-Pana-sati*" meditation in Buddhism. If you are a trained meditator, or if you can improve your mindfulness up to this advanced level, you will be benefited from the next stages of *"Ana-Pana-sati"* meditation.

In conclusion,

To sum up, in simple terms, mindfulness is having a moment by moment awareness of one's experience without judgment. Practicing mindfulness meditation is a way of cultivating mindfulness.

The *"Satipatthana Sutta"* is the text that contains the Lord Buddha's teachings on practicing mindfulness meditation. It is thought to be the foundation for the modern concepts of practicing mindfulness meditation.

At first, practicing mindfulness meditation may look difficult. It certainly is. However, you can start to be mindful when you are doing small day to day chores at home, and then switch to the meditation practices like *"Ana-Pana-sati"* meditation. If you do this right, you will be able to see the results very soon.

Strategy No.3 Practicing a Relaxation Exercise

If you are a fitness geek, or if you think I need some sort of exercise with some sort of a goal like weight loss or getting into good shape, etc. this would be a better way of managing stress.

However, there are some instances that some of us face a situation where we feel like we can't hold things together. Though we want to go to the gym, the laziness overrides our ambition of achieving our goals, or the extreme stress drives us to stay at home, or postpone our fitness goals.

Practicing a relaxation exercise is a good way of cultivating mindfulness as well. As we discussed in the previous chapter, there are various methods like "Tai Chi", "Yoga", etc. can give you the benefits of extra toning of your muscles at the same time you achieve a clear, and healthy mind.

In this chapter, we will be discussing Practicing Yoga as a way of managing stress. Most of you may know the physical benefits of practicing Yoga, but I will explain the basic outline of what is Yoga and its other benefits.

Practicing Yoga as a Relaxation Exercise

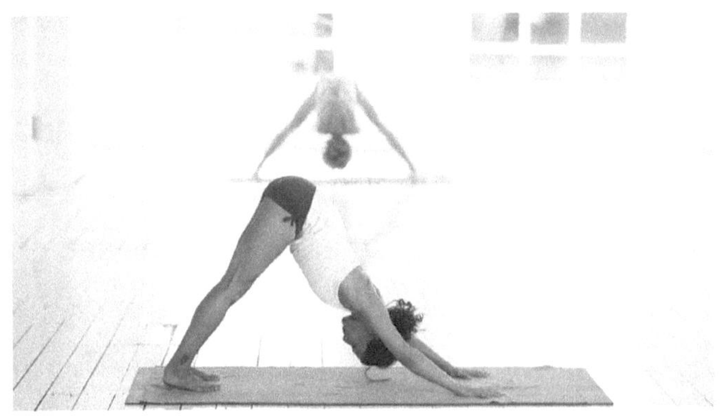

What is Yoga?

The word "Yoga" originates from Sanskrit and means "to join, to unite". Yoga is a way of living that aims towards a healthy mind in a healthy body. Thus, yoga exercises promote not only a balanced development of man's physical health but also mental, and spiritual wellbeing as well.

History of Yoga

Historically, a character who lived in India whose name was "Patanjali" is thought to be the founder of yoga. He had his work based on medicine, grammar, and yoga. All of these together cover the body, spirit, and intellect of an individual.

He named these as "Yoga Sutras". According to his teachings, there are 8 limbs of yoga sutras. More descriptively, they are mentioned below.

1. "Yama"

These are aimed at creating a better world. That is to say, not harming anyone, or anything, truthfulness, non-stealing, being a non-grasping attitude, and living a godly life are the main five universal truths of life.

2. "Niyama"

These are five personal disciplines that help to increase one's inner peace. In other words, cleanliness, contentedness, self-discipline, dedication to god, and lastly self-study and study of scriptures.

3. "Asana"

Asanas are the various postures of yoga. Devoted and continuous practicing of above will lead to the physical wellbeing of a person.

4. "Pranayama"

This is the practice of breath control techniques.

5. "Pratyahara"

This means that achieving a state of a non-attached attitude of body, and mind. Certainly, this would give a person a less stressful, and peaceful mental state.

6. "Dharana"

This is increasing the level of concentration of a person. This aims at being able to hold on to a subject mentally.

7. "Dhyana"

Dhyana is meditation. In other words, developing a quiet mindful, and meditative state.

8. "Samadhi"

This is achieving a state of bliss. Above all, once you properly practice yoga, you will feel reaching a state of divine.

Most importantly, when we study the teachings of "Patanjali" it is obvious that one can achieve a good level of physical fitness while achieving mental and spiritual wellbeing as well.

That is why yoga is nowadays very popular among lots of people as a mode of relieving stress and keeping a good healthy, fit lifestyle.

Practicing Yoga for a Healthy Life – Benefits of Yoga

Yoga asanas Build Strength, Flexibility, and Toning of Muscles.

There are a variety of asanas that anyone can master easily. These include standing poses, sitting poses, supine and prone poses.

Besides, some twisting poses and inverted poses need more practice and experience.

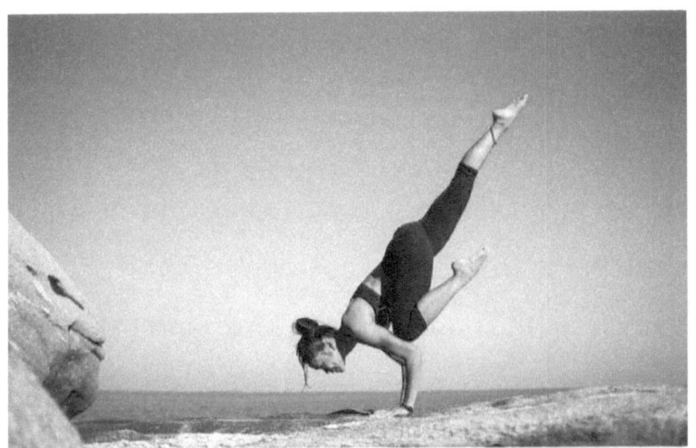

Yoga asanas promote both physical and mental health. But there are different types of yoga poses that need more practice, and experience.

When you practice these poses repetitively with self-discipline, you will experience that your body adapts to them. At the same time, it builds your muscles increasing their flexibility, strengthening them, and toning them.

Additionally, these exercises will help you to lose weight and have a perfect shaped body as well. So, girls, if you want a perfect figure, try some yoga!

However, practicing yoga might seem like just stretching. But it can do much more for your body from the way you feel, look, and move.

It Improves Respiration, Energy, and Vitality

These asanas come with stretching of muscles but at the same time, you have to practice breathing techniques. Eventually, by properly mastering these breathing techniques will aid your respiration and vitality.

Furthermore, you will feel more energetic, and more relaxed as yoga has the power to remove toxins from your body as well as keep your blood circulation, and other biological processes function smoothly.

Further, these will increase the body's power of self-healing as well.

Helps in Attention, Focus, and Concentration

While you are practicing asanas and breathing techniques, you need to have the proper concentration to make them work properly. Some of the inverted poses need real-time concentration and balance.

Therefore, by practicing yoga you will develop attention, focus, and concentration.

You may be a student, and you may need to learn and remember things easily. Therefore, this would be a great step in your life!

Reduces Stress and Tension both Physically and Mentally

Most importantly, when you are practicing yoga poses, with time, and experience you will achieve greater concentration. So, you will be able to perform more, and more.

This will give you a relaxed feeling while taking away any negative thoughts you have. Moreover, it pushes you into a meditative state while performing those poses with great care and concentration.

Subsequently, this will achieve a great mental power making you handle any sort of mental stress, and keep you away from depression.

Certainly, building muscular strength and flexibility reduces tension on your joints, etc.

and helps you in diseases like osteoarthritis too.

Enhances Personal Power and Let You have Better Relationships

Above all, practicing yoga will make you a better person. Meanwhile, the non-attached attitude drives you into a meditative state teaching you to live in harmony with others.

The confidence you develop by practicing difficult yoga poses will enhance your power. So, you will achieve a better place in the society you live on.

The ultimate result is that you will become a better person who can build good relationships with others.

Conclusion

To sum up, Yoga exercises promote the physical, mental, and social wellbeing of a person.

It helps to improve your muscle strength, manage stress, and anxiety, and keeps you relaxing. Likewise, it helps you achieve good relationships.

Practicing yoga for a healthy life comes with self-discipline, and regular practicing of your yoga poses.

Summary

The 3 strategies mentioned in this book are easy to implement at home. In the beginning, you can practice these principles alone but when you improve yourself, you may need a helping hand.

For instance, although you can practice simple yoga poses at first, you may need the help of a yoga instructor to practice more complex twisting, and inverted poses later. Likewise, you may be able to master the initial stages of the mindfulness meditation, but you may need an instructor at the later stages of meditation.

Above all, managing stress could be a choice that we can make in our lifestyles. The way you arrange your life, and its decisions can make a great impact on how you face stressful situations in life. Not any other person, but YOU can heal yourself. When you throw away the negative feelings, and thoughts like greediness, hatred, desire, ignorance, you will feel a great difference in your life. By doing this, not only yourself but also the people around you will reap these benefits too.

Let's make a better world!

The End.

About the Author

Dr. Pasindu Abeysundara is a medical practitioner from Sri Lanka. He is interested in sharing his knowledge in medicine to the general public in a simplified and easy to understand manner. Further, he believes in the prevention of disease is better than cure.

He was graduated from the University of Peradeniya in Sri Lanka with an MBBS degree and has the experience of treating patients in the fields of Medicine, Surgery, and Psychiatry for years in various parts of Sri Lanka.

To visit his website, type the following on your web browser.

https://healthfactsbydoctorpasindu.com/

Other Books by the Author

To visit the Author Central page on Amazon,
type the following in your web browser.

amazon.com/author/pasindu-abeysundara

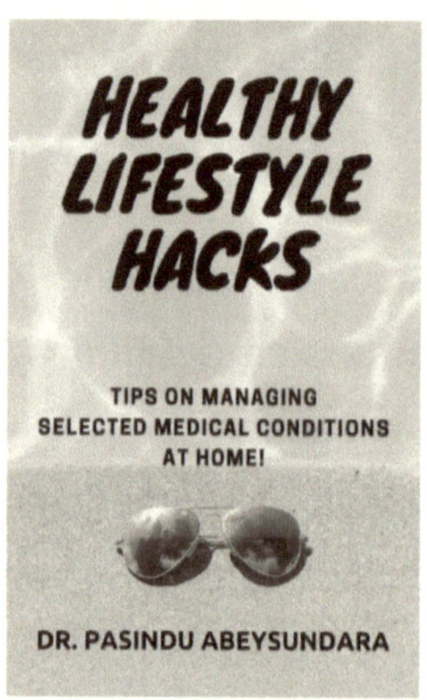

Healthy Lifestyle Hacks

Topics covered in this book are,

Chapter 1. How to Treat a LIGAMENT SPRAIN at Home!

Chapter 2. How to Treat the UPPER BACK PAIN due to RHOMBOID SPASMS at Home!

Chapter 3. How to Treat DRY EYES at Home!

Chapter 4. How to Treat the HEEL PAIN due to PLANTAR FASCIITIS, at Home!

Chapter 5. How to TAKE CARE of a BEDBOUND PERSON at Home!

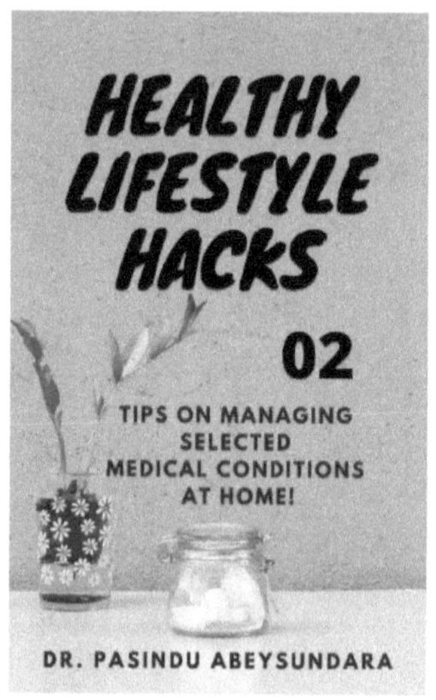

Topics covered in this book are;

One Last Thing!

If you enjoyed this book or found it to be useful, I would be grateful if you could post a short review on Amazon. Your support does make a big difference. And I read all the reviews personally so I can get your feedback and make this writing experience even better.

If you would like to leave a review, then all you need to do is click the review button link on this book's page on Amazon.

Thanks again for your support!

Dr. Pasindu Abeysundara.